PowerPhonics™

Visiting the Vet:

Learning the V Sound

Janet Carson

The Rosen Publishing Group's
PowerKids Press™
New York

Our dog Val has hurt her leg.

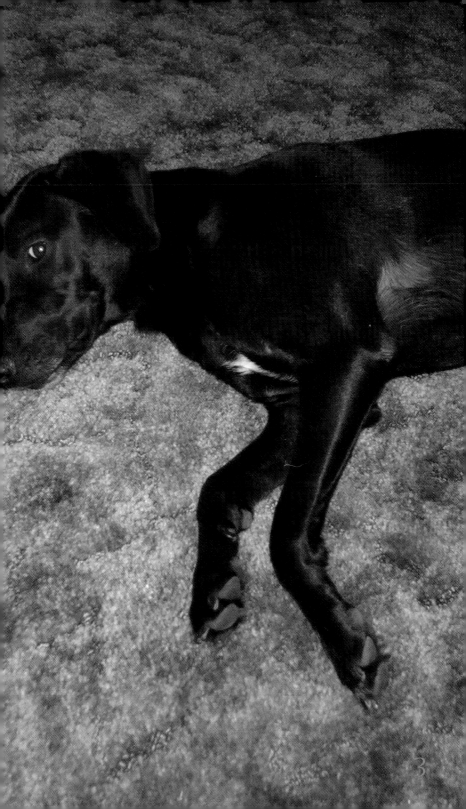

We take Val to the vet in our van.

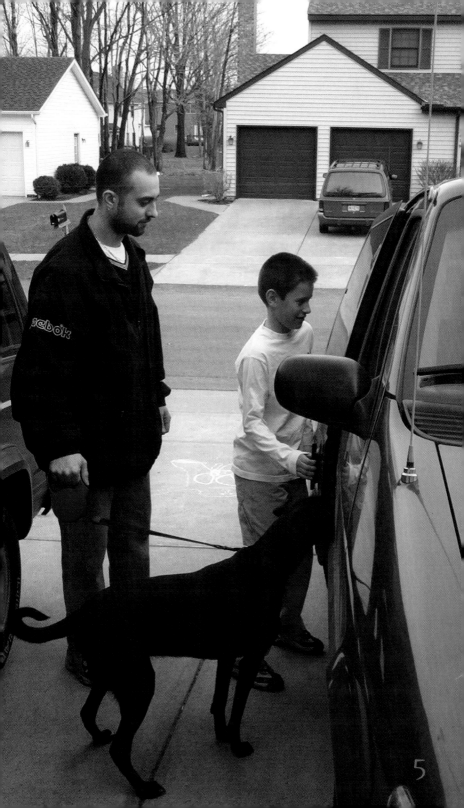

We wait with Val to visit the vet.

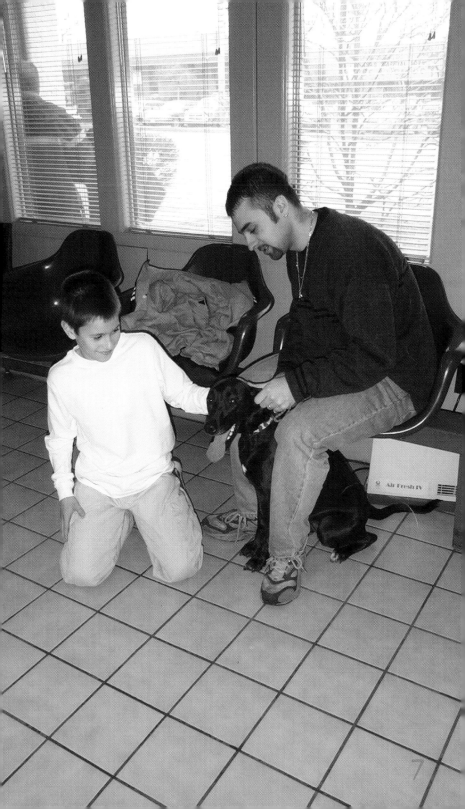

We see a cat that will visit the vet.

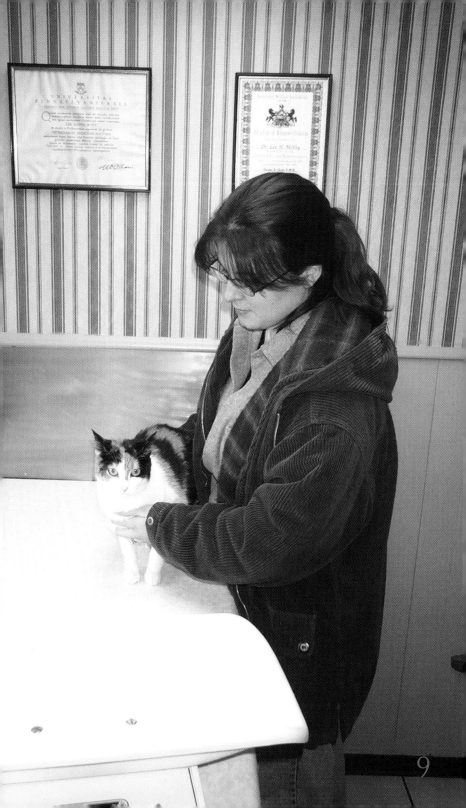

We see a bunny that will visit the vet.

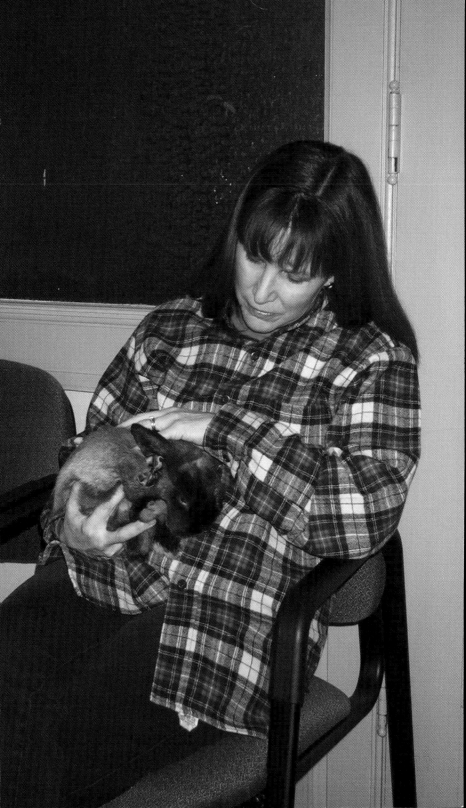

Val is next to visit the vet.

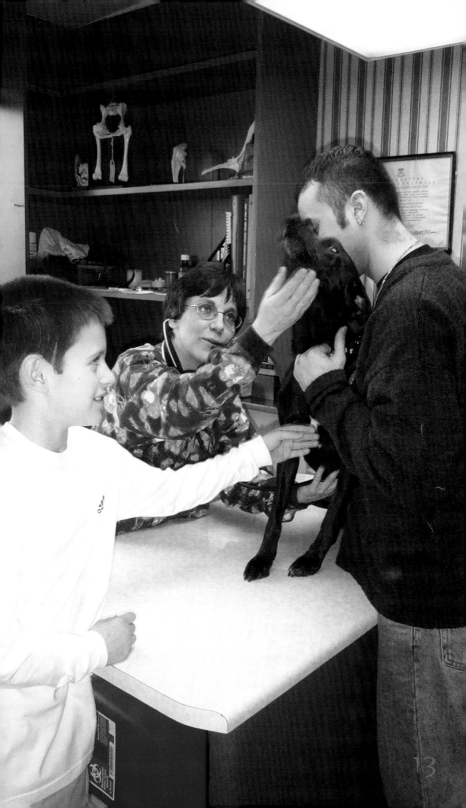

The vet looks at Val's leg.

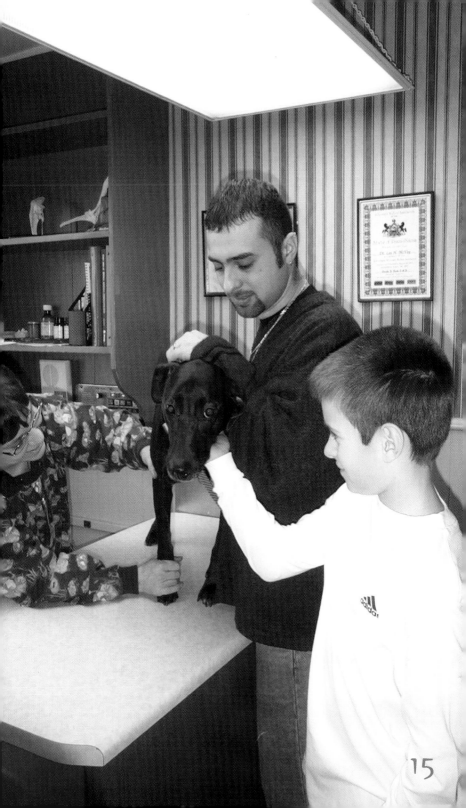

The vet helps Val feel better.

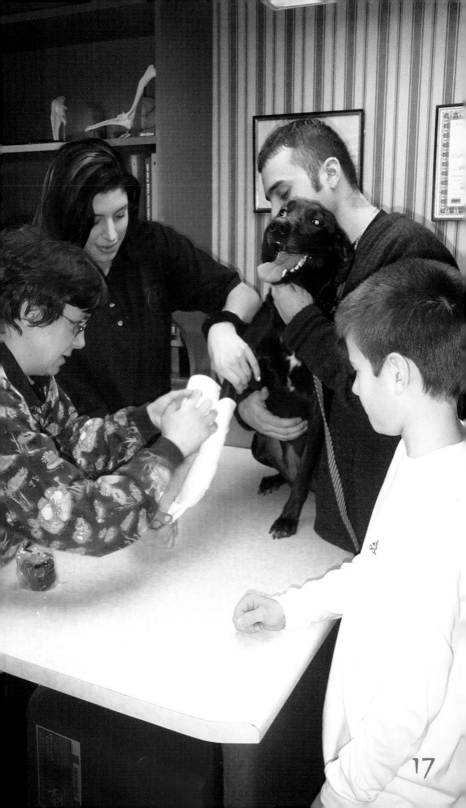

The vet says that Val will be O.K.

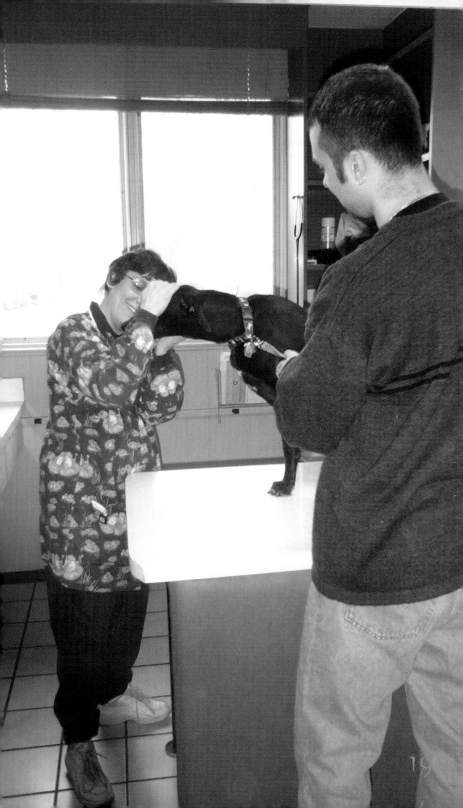

The vet says good-bye to Val.

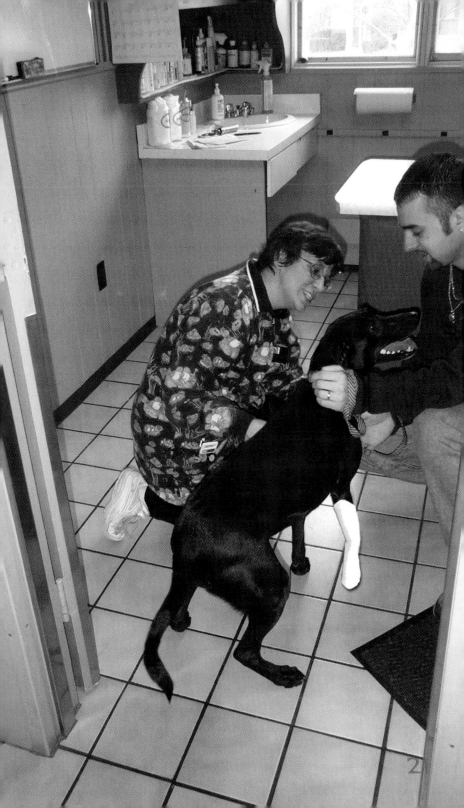

Word List

Val

van

vet

visit

Instructional Guide

Note to Instructors:

One of the essential skills that enable a young child to read is the ability to associate letter-sound symbols and blend these sounds to form words. Phonics instruction can teach children a system that will help them decode unfamiliar words and, in turn, enhance their word-recognition skills. We offer a phonics-based series of books that are easy to read and understand. Each book pairs words and pictures that reinforce specific phonetic sounds in a logical sequence. Topics are based on curriculum goals appropriate for early readers in the areas of science, social studies, and health.

Letter/Sound: v – Say the following words: *family, valentine, vase.* Have the child name two words that have the same beginning sound. Continue with: *van, fed, vote; fan, very, vat; vine, vest, for; visit, vet, fine.* As the child responds, list the initial **v** words on a chalkboard or dry-erase board. Have the child contribute additional initial **v** words to the list. Have them underline the consonant **v** in each word.

Phonics Activities: List the following words on the chalkboard or dry-erase board and have the child decode them: *man, get, pine, pal, cat, rest.* Have the child write a rhyming word that begins with **v** for each word. Remind them to use capital **V** for names of people. Have the child use a pair of the rhyming words in a single sentence. (Example: *A man can drive a van.*)

- Play "Vanishing Vs." Have the child color and/or cut from magazines pictures of items with the initial **v** sound. Mount and label the pictures and arrange them on a table. In addition, list the initial **v** words on the chalkboard or dry-erase board. To play the game, have the child close their eyes while a word is erased from the list. Have the child name the missing word and locate its picture. Encourage them to use complete sentences, such as, *The vacuum cleaner has vanished.* After practice, vary the game by removing pictures and having the child point to the word that names the Vanished **V** item.

- Have the child tell whether they hear the **v** sound at the beginning or end of each of the following words: *vase, very, vote, van, cave, live, gave, five,* etc. As the child responds, list the words in two columns according to the position of the consonant **v**.

Additional Resources:

- Flanagan, Alice K. *Dr. Friedman Helps Animals.* Danbury, CT: Children's Press, 2000.
- Kunhardt, Edith. *I'm Going to Be a Vet.* New York: Scholastic, Inc., 1996.
- Leonard, Marcia. *The Pet Vet.* Brookfield, CT: Millbrook Press, Inc., 1999.

Many thanks to Dr. P. J. Polumbo and the staff at
Glenwood Pet Hospital for their help and cooperation.

Published in 2002 by The Rosen Publishing Group, Inc.
29 East 21st Street, New York, NY 10010

Book Design: Ron A. Churley

Photo Credits: Cover, pp. 3, 5, 7, 11, 13, 15, 17, 19, 21 by Karey L.
Schuckers-Churley; p. 9 by Ron A. Churley.

Library of Congress Cataloging-in-Publication Data

Carson, Janet.
  Visiting the vet : learning the V sound / Janet Carson.—1st ed.
     p. cm. — (Power phonics/phonics for the real world)
  ISBN 0-8239-5934-1 (lib. bdg.)
  ISBN 0-8239-8279-3 (pbk.)
  6 pack ISBN 0-8239-9247-0
  1. Veterinary medicine—Juvenile literature. 2. Veterinary
hospitals—Juvenile literature. 3. Veterinarians—Juvenile literature.
  4. English language—Consonants—Juvenile literature. [1. Veterinary
hospitals. 2. Veterinarians. 3. English language—Consonants.] I. Title.
II. Series.
  SF756 .C37 2001
  636.089—dc21

                                        2001000780

Manufactured in the United States of America